The Scope of Practice

FOR ACADEMIC NURSE EDUCATORS

2012 REVISION

National League for Nursing
Certification Commission
Certification Test Development Committee

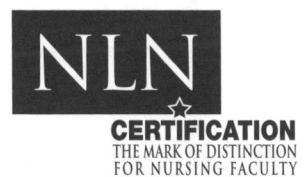

NLN

★

CERTIFICATION
THE MARK OF DISTINCTION
FOR NURSING FACULTY

National League for Nursing
61 Broadway New York, NY 10006
www.nln.org

First printing 2005. Revised 2012.

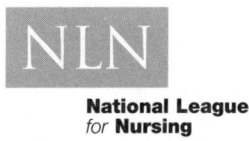

National League
for **Nursing**

ISBN: 978-1-934758-17-5

Printed in The United Sates of America

9

DRC1117

Table of Contents

Introduction

The purpose of this document is to describe academic nursing education as a specialty area and an advanced nursing practice role within professional nursing. *The Scope of Practice for Academic Nurse Educators 2012 Revision* outlines the definition, historical perspective, values and beliefs, theoretical framework, scope of practice, and competencies or standards of practice of academic nursing education.

The Scope of Practice for Academic Nurse Educators was first developed by the National League for Nursing's Certification Governance Committee and published by the NLN in 2005. At that time, the leadership of the National League for Nursing and the members of the committee believed that recognition of academic nursing education as a specialty and an advanced nursing practice role was essential and that a description of the scope and competencies of nurse educator practice and a certification exam linked to those competencies was required.

In 2010 and 2011, the National League for Nursing Certification Commission collaborated to perform an updated nurse educator practice analysis. This systematic practice analysis assessment was intended to identify any changes in the job-related responsibilities of individuals who fulfill the full scope of the nurse faculty role. The results of the 2010-2011 practice analysis resulted in slight revisions to the nurse educator certification test blueprint.

Both the 2005 version and the revised 2012 version of *The Scope of Practice for Academic Nurse Educators* are aligned and consistent with the pattern of documents with which the nursing community is familiar, namely *Nursing: Scope and Standards of Practice* Second Edition (American Nurses Association, 2010), and *Scope and Standards of Practice for Nursing Professional Development* (American Nurses Association, 2000).

Definition

Academic nursing education is the process of facilitating learning through curriculum design, teaching, evaluation, advisement, and other activities undertaken by faculty in schools of nursing. Academic nursing education is a specialty area and an advanced practice role within professional nursing.

Academic nurse educators engage in a number of roles and functions, each of which reflects the core competencies of nursing faculty (see pp. 14-19). The extent to which a specific nurse educator implements these competencies varies according to many factors, including the mission of the nurse educator's institution, the nurse educator's rank, the nurse educator's academic preparation, and the type of program in which the nurse educator teaches.

Nursing education takes place in diverse settings that include, but are not limited to, technical schools, hospitals, two-year colleges, four-year colleges, and universities. The implementation of the academic faculty role may occur in traditional classroom-based environments as well as in non-traditional environments.

Historical Perspective

The development of educational programs for the preparation of nurses parallels the evolution of nursing as a distinct profession requiring a specialized body of knowledge and skills. One of the earliest known nurse training programs was the Deaconess Institute established in Kaiserwerth, Germany, in 1836. Deaconesses were women who promised to work for Christ by teaching or nursing. The institute became well known, and graduates of the program spread the Kaiserwerth model of care of the ill and infirm throughout the world (Donahue, 1996).

Florence Nightingale trained at the Kaiserwerth Institute in 1851. On her return to England from Crimea in 1856, Nightingale set about achieving her two key goals: "reform of army sanitary practices and the establishment of a school for nurses" (Kalisch and Kalisch, 1995, p. 36). Today, Nightingale is credited with defining a theoretical foundation for the practice of nursing and founding the first independent, organized training program for nurses (Donahue, 1996).

In the United States, the mid-nineteenth century saw calls for formal training of nurses by organizations such as the American Medical Association. The first training school for nurses in America was established in 1872 at the New England Hospital.

By 1902, there were 492 schools of nursing in the United States. Training programs expected strict discipline, long hours, and a strong focus on learning through practice. Programs began to expand from two to three years in length and schools known for their high quality of training attracted students of increasing caliber. In 1905, Bellevue Hospital had 2000 applicants (Kalisch and Kalisch, 1995).

During the early twentieth century, most nurses were prepared in hospital-based programs. However, starting with the University of Minnesota in 1909, collegiate settings became the locus for programs of registered nursing education at the undergraduate and graduate levels. The approach to providing registered nursing education in community colleges was developed by Dr. Mildred Montag in 1949.

During this period and beyond, several important studies guided the evolution of nursing education. In 1923, the first evaluation of nursing education, by Goldmark, was published. Examples of other key documents include: *Nurses, Patients, and Pocketbooks* (1923), *Nursing Schools Today and Tomorrow* (1934), *Nursing for the Future* (1948), *Nurses for a Growing Nation* (1957), *Toward Quality in Nursing*

(1961), *American Nurses Association Position Paper on Education for Nursing* (1965), and *Extending the Scope of Nursing Practice* (1971) (Kalisch & Kalisch, 1995). These documents provided important guidance to the development of nursing education in the United States and Canada.

As nursing progressed to become a profession, the science of nursing was further delineated and the body of knowledge and skills unique to generalist and advanced practice nursing was developed and refined. Preparation of professional nurses transitioned from "training" to "education."

The first organization for nursing in the United States was officially developed in 1893. The American Society of Superintendents of Training Schools of Nurses (ASSTSN)* was formed for "the establishment and maintenance of a universal standard of training" for nursing (Fondiller, 1999).

The first formal training programs for practical nurses were started by the Brooklyn, New York YMCA in 1893; however, the first school was not organized until 1897.

The shortage of nurses that followed World War II prompted the expansion of practical nurse (PN) programs, with most housed in public schools. The practical nurse programs of today are commonly one year in length, and most PN education takes place in vocational/technical schools and community colleges (Kelly & Joel, 1996).

Although nursing education has existed for more than 160 years, academic nursing education as a specialty area of practice with a defined theoretical basis, body of knowledge, and certification has been slow to develop. Preparation of nurses as educators has occurred in graduate programs of nursing or education or through continuing education, mentoring, or experience. In order to further advance nursing education, new models of research-based nursing education must emerge. The precedent of relying on tradition and past practices must be replaced with proposed changes emanating from "evidence that substantiates the science of nursing education and provides the foundation for best educational practices" (National League for Nursing, 2005b, p. 1).

The ASSTSN evolved into the National League for Nursing Education (NLNE) in 1912 and then the National League for Nursing (NLN) in 1952.

Values and Beliefs

Academic nurse educators believe that education is a self-actualizing, creative, lifetime endeavor involving values clarification, progressive systematic inquiry, critical analysis, and judgment.

As a distinct specialty of advanced nursing practice, academic nursing education has a set of defined values and beliefs. They are evident in the *NLN's Hallmarks of Excellence in Nursing Education*© (outlined below) and are incorporated into the standards of practice.

NLN'S HALLMARKS OF EXCELLENCE IN NURSING EDUCATION©

Students

Students are excited about learning, exhibit a spirit of inquiry and a sense of wonderment, and commit to lifelong learning.

Students are committed to innovation, continuous quality/performance improvement, and excellence.

Students are committed to a career in nursing.

Faculty

The faculty complement includes a cadre of individuals who have expertise as educators, clinicians, and, as is relevant to the institution's mission, researchers.

The unique contributions of each faculty member in helping the program achieve its goals are valued, rewarded, and recognized.

Faculty members are accountable for promoting excellence and providing leadership in their area(s) of expertise.

Faculty model a commitment to lifelong learning, involvement in professional nursing associations, and nursing as a career.

All faculty have structured preparation for the faculty role, as well as competence in their area(s) of teaching responsibility.

Continuous Quality Improvement

The program engages in a variety of activities that promote excellence, including accreditation from national nursing accreditation bodies.

The program design, implementation, and evaluation are continuously reviewed and revised to achieve and maintain excellence.

Curriculum

The curriculum is flexible and reflects current societal and health care trends and issues, research findings and innovative practices, as well as local and global perspectives.

The curriculum provides experiential cultural learning activities that enhance students' abilities to think critically, reflect thoughtfully, and provide culturally-sensitive, evidence-based nursing care to diverse populations.

The curriculum emphasizes students' values development, socialization to the new role, commitment to lifelong learning, and creativity.

The curriculum provides learning experiences that prepare graduates to assume roles that are essential to quality nursing practice, including but not limited to roles of care provider, patient advocate, teacher, communicator, change agent, care coordinator, user of information technology, collaborator, and decision maker.

The curriculum provides learning experiences that support evidence-based practice, multidisciplinary approaches to care, student achievement of clinical competence, and, as appropriate, expertise in a specialty role.

The curriculum is evidence-based.

Teaching/Learning/Evaluation Strategies

Teaching/learning/evaluation strategies are innovative and varied to facilitate and enhance learning by a diverse student population.

Teaching/learning/evaluation strategies promote collegial dialogue and interaction between and among faculty, students, and colleagues in nursing and other professions.

Teaching/learning/evaluation strategies used by faculty are evidence-based.

Resources

Partnerships in which the program is engaged promote excellence in nursing education, enhance the profession, benefit the community, and expand service/learning opportunities.

Technology is used effectively to support teaching/learning/evaluation processes.

Student support services are culturally-sensitive, innovative, and empower students during the recruitment, retention, progression, graduation, and career planning processes.

Financial resources of the program are used to support curriculum innovation, visionary long-range planning, faculty development, an empowering learning environment, creative initiatives, continuous quality improvement of the program, and evidence-based teaching/learning/evaluation practices.

Innovation

The design and implementation of the program is innovative and seeks to build on traditional approaches to nursing education.

The innovativeness of the program helps to create a preferred future for nursing.

Educational Research

Faculty and students contribute to the development of the science of nursing education through the critique, utilization, dissemination or conduct of research.

Faculty and students explore the impact of student learning experiences on the health of the communities they serve.

Environment

The educational environment empowers students and faculty and promotes collegial dialogue, innovation, change, creativity, values development, and ethical behavior.

Leadership

Faculty, students, and alumni are respected as leaders in the parent organization, as well as in local, state, regional, national, or international communities.

Faculty, students, and alumni are prepared for and assume leadership roles that advance quality nursing care; promote positive change, innovation, and excellence; and enhance the power and influence of the nursing profession.

Theoretical Foundations

Nursing's Social Policy Statement: The Essence of the Profession (American Nurses Association, 2010) builds on previous work and provides the following contemporary definition of nursing: "Nursing is the protection, promotion, and optimization of health and abilities, prevention of illness and injury, alleviation of suffering through the diagnosis and treatment of human response, and advocacy in the care of individuals, families, communities, and populations" (American Nurses Association, 2010, p. 3).

As a specialty area of advanced nursing practice, academic nursing education has a theoretical foundation that includes models and theories from nursing science, "educational psychology, instructional technology, instructional design, tests and measurement, and evaluation theory" (Caputi & Engelmann, 2004, p. 3).

Several models and theories have been used to develop the scope and standards of practice in the academic nurse educator role that are relevant to faculty teaching in all types of nursing programs: practical nurse, associate degree, diploma, baccalaureate, master's, and doctoral. Examples of models and theories from education with relevance for nursing education include Boyer's Scholarship of Engagement (Boyer, 1990), Kolb's Learning Cycle (Kolb, 1984), Bloom's taxonomy of learning objectives (Krathwol, Bloom, & Masia, 1964), learning theories such as Knowles's adult learning theory (Knowles, Holton, & Swanson, 1998), community-academic partnerships (Tagliareni & Marck, 1997), and service-learning (Community Campus Partnerships for Health, 2004).

Boyer (1990) described a perspective of the scholarly role of faculty that went beyond the traditional interpretation of research as the "only way to increase the knowledge of the discipline and as the only means for incentive and compensation of the academic professional" (Kirkpatrick & Valley, 2004). He outlined four types of scholarship in which faculty engage: discovery (disciplined investigative efforts leading to new knowledge), integration (synthesis, making connections across disciplines), application (using knowledge in implementing a practice role or in service to the larger community), and teaching (transmitting, transforming, and extending knowledge). The extent to which a particular academic nurse educator engages in each type of scholarship will vary in accord with factors such as the nurse educator's professional goals and the type of program in which the nurse educator teaches.

Scope of Practice

"The scope of practice statement describes the 'who, what, where, when, why, and how' of nursing practice." (American Nurses Association, 2004, p. 1). The term "academic nurse educator" refers to an individual who fulfills a faculty role in an academic setting. In nursing, this role is implemented in practical nurse (PN), registered nurse (RN), and graduate programs.

Whereas individuals with appointments to a nursing faculty may hold advanced preparation in disciplines supportive to nursing (e.g., nutrition, pharmacology), the scope of practice described here relates to individuals with advanced preparation in nursing who teach nursing courses. "Competence as an educator can be established, recognized, and expanded through master's and/or doctoral education, post-master's certificate programs, continuing professional development, mentoring activities, and professional certification as a faculty member." (National League for Nursing, 2002, p. 4).

Nursing education takes place in diverse settings which include, but are not limited to, technical schools, hospitals, two-year colleges, four-year colleges, and universities. The implementation of the academic faculty role may occur in traditional classroom-based environments or in non-traditional environments.

Academic nurse educators engage in a number of roles and functions, each of which reflects the core competencies of nursing faculty. Those competencies include the following: 1) facilitate learning, 2) facilitate learner development and socialization, 3) use assessment and evaluation strategies, 4) participate in curriculum design and evaluation of program outcomes, 5) function as a change agent and leader, 6) pursue continuous quality improvement in the nurse educator role, 7) engage in scholarship, and 8) function within the educational environment.

The extent to which a specific nurse educator implements these competencies varies according to many factors, including the mission of the nurse educator's institution, the nurse educator's rank, the nurse educator's academic preparation, and the type of program in which the nurse educator teaches.

The development of a master nurse educator evolves over time. To that end, it is recognized that many nurse educators function at a competent level early in their careers, but mastery occurs with guidance, ongoing professional development, and practice.

Standards of Practice

Standards of practice describe the responsibilities for which nurses in a particular role are accountable (American Nurses Association, 2010). For academic nurse educators, those responsibilities relate to the eight core competencies outlined by the National League for Nursing. They are as follows:

CORE COMPETENCIES OF NURSE EDUCATORS© WITH TASK STATEMENTS

Competency I: Facilitate Learning

Nurse educators are responsible for creating an environment in classroom, laboratory, and clinical settings that facilitates student learning and the achievement of desired cognitive, affective, and psychomotor outcomes. To facilitate learning effectively, the nurse educator:

- Implements a variety of teaching strategies appropriate to learner needs, desired learner outcomes, content, and context

- Grounds teaching strategies in educational theory and evidence-based teaching practices

- Recognizes multicultural, gender, and experiential influences on teaching and learning

- Engages in self-reflection and continued learning to improve teaching practices that facilitate learning

- Uses information technologies skillfully to support the teaching-learning process

- Practices skilled oral, written, and electronic communication that reflects an awareness of self and others, along with an ability to convey ideas in a variety of contexts

- Models critical and reflective thinking

- Creates opportunities for learners to develop their critical thinking and critical reasoning skills

- Shows enthusiasm for teaching, learning, and nursing that inspires and motivates students

- Demonstrates interest in and respect for learners

- Uses personal attributes (e.g., caring, confidence, patience, integrity, and flexibility) that facilitate learning

- Develops collegial working relationships with students, faculty colleagues, and clinical agency personnel to promote positive learning environments

- Maintains the professional practice knowledge base needed to help learners prepare for contemporary nursing practice

- Serves as a role model of professional nursing

Competency II: Facilitate Learner Development and Socialization

Nurse educators recognize their responsibility for helping students develop as nurses and integrate the values and behaviors expected of those who fulfill that role. To facilitate learner development and socialization effectively, the nurse educator:

- Identifies individual learning styles and unique learning needs of international, adult, multicultural, educationally disadvantaged, physically challenged, at-risk, and second degree learners

- Provides resources to diverse learners that help meet their individual learning needs

- Engages in effective advisement and counseling strategies that help learners meet their professional goals

- Creates learning environments that are focused on socialization to the role of the nurse and facilitate learners' self-reflection and personal goal setting

- Fosters the cognitive, psychomotor, and affective development of learners

- Recognizes the influence of teaching styles and interpersonal interactions on learner outcomes

- Assists learners to develop the ability to engage in thoughtful and constructive self and peer evaluation

- Models professional behaviors for learners including, but not limited to, involvement in professional organizations, engagement in lifelong learning activities, dissemination of information through publications and presentations, and advocacy

Competency III: Use Assessment and Evaluation Strategies

Nurse educators use a variety of strategies to assess and evaluate student learning in classroom, laboratory and clinical settings, as well as in all domains of learning. To use assessment and evaluation strategies effectively, the nurse educator:

- Uses extant literature to develop evidence-based assessment and evaluation practices

- Uses a variety of strategies to assess and evaluate learning in the cognitive, psychomotor, and affective domains

- Implements evidence-based assessment and evaluation strategies that are appropriate to the learner and to learning goals

- Uses assessment and evaluation data to enhance the teaching-learning process

- Provides timely, constructive, and thoughtful feedback to learners

- Demonstrates skill in the design and use of tools for assessing clinical practice

Competency IV: Participate in Curriculum Design and Evaluation of Program Outcomes

Nurse educators are responsible for formulating program outcomes and designing curricula that reflect contemporary health care trends and prepare graduates to function effectively in the health care environment. To participate effectively in curriculum design and systematic evaluation of program outcomes, the nurse educator:

- Ensures that the curriculum reflects institutional philosophy and mission, current nursing and health care trends, and community and societal needs so as to prepare graduates for practice in a complex, dynamic, multicultural health care environment

- Demonstrates knowledge of curriculum development including identifying program outcomes, developing competency statements, writing learning objectives, and selecting appropriate learning activities and evaluation strategies

- Bases curriculum design and implementation decisions on sound educational principles, theory and research

- Revises the curriculum based on assessment of program outcomes, learner needs, and societal and health care trends

- Implements curricular revisions using appropriate change theories and strategies

- Creates and maintains community and clinical partnerships that support educational goals

- Collaborates with external constituencies throughout the process of curriculum revision

- Designs and implements program assessment models that promote continuous quality improvement of all aspects of the program

Competency V: Function as a Change Agent and Leader

Nurse educators function as change agents and leaders to create a preferred future for nursing education and nursing practice. To function effectively as a change agent and leader, the nurse educator:

- Models cultural sensitivity when advocating for change

- Integrates a long-term, innovative, and creative perspective into the nurse educator role

- Participates in interdisciplinary efforts to address health care and educational needs locally, regionally, nationally, or internationally

- Evaluates organizational effectiveness in nursing education

- Implements strategies for organizational change

- Provides leadership in the parent institution as well as in the nursing program to enhance the visibility of nursing and its contributions to the academic community

- Promotes innovative practices in educational environments

- Develops leadership skills to shape and implement change

Competency VI: Pursue Continuous Quality Improvement in the Nurse Educator Role

Nurse educators recognize that their role is multidimensional and that an ongoing commitment to develop and maintain competence in the role is essential. To pursue continuous quality improvement in the nurse educator role, the individual:

- Demonstrates a commitment to life-long learning

- Recognizes that career enhancement needs and activities change as experience is gained in the role

- Participates in professional development opportunities that increase one's effectiveness in the role

- Balances the teaching, scholarship, and service demands inherent in the role of educator and member of an academic institution

- Uses feedback gained from self, peer, student, and administrative evaluation to improve role effectiveness

- Engages in activities that promote one's socialization to the role

- Uses knowledge of legal and ethical issues relevant to higher education and nursing education as a basis for influencing, designing, and implementing policies and procedures related to students, faculty, and the educational environment

- Mentors and supports faculty colleagues

Competency VII: Engage in Scholarship

Nurse educators acknowledge that scholarship is an integral component of the faculty role, and that teaching itself is a scholarly activity. To engage effectively in scholarship, the nurse educator:

- Draws on extant literature to design evidence-based teaching and evaluation practices

- Exhibits a spirit of inquiry about teaching and learning, student development, evaluation methods, and other aspects of the role

- Designs and implements scholarly activities in an established area of expertise

- Disseminates nursing and teaching knowledge to a variety of audiences through various means

- Demonstrates skill in proposal writing for initiatives that include, but are not limited to, research, resource acquisition, program development, and policy development

- Demonstrates qualities of a scholar: integrity, courage, perseverance, vitality, and creativity

Competency VIII. Function within the Educational Environment

Nurse educators are knowledgeable about the educational environment within which they practice and recognize how political, institutional, social, and economic forces impact their role. To function as a good "citizen of the academy," the nurse educator:

- Uses knowledge of history and current trends and issues in higher education as a basis for making recommendations and decisions on educational issues

- Identifies how social, economic, political, and institutional forces influence higher education in general and nursing education in particular

- Develops networks, collaborations, and partnerships to enhance nursing's influence within the academic community

- Determines own professional goals within the context of academic nursing and the mission of the parent institution and nursing program

- Integrates the values of respect, collegiality, professionalism, and caring to build an organizational climate that fosters the development of students and teachers

- Incorporates the goals of the nursing program and the mission of the parent institution when proposing change or managing issues

- Assumes a leadership role in various levels of institutional governance

- Advocates for nursing and nursing education in the political arena

Note: The original competencies were developed in 2005 by the NLN's Task Group on Nurse Educator Competencies. The following professionals served as members of the 2005 Task Group:

Judith A. Halstead, DNS, RN (Chair)

Wanda Bonnel, PhD, RN

Barbara Chamberlain, MSN, RN, CNS, C, CCRN

Pauline M. Green, PhD, RN

Karolyn R. Hanna, PhD, RN

Carol Heinrich, PhD, RN

Barbara Patterson, PhD, RN

Helen Speziale, EdD, RN

Elizabeth Stokes, EdD, RN

Jane Sumner, PhD, RN

Cesarina Thompson, PhD, RN

Diane M. Tomasic, EdD, RN

Patricia Young, PhD, RN

Mary Anne Rizzolo, EdD, RN, FAAN, (NLN Staff Liaison)

The Scope of Practice for Academic Nurse Educators (2005) was developed by the NLN's Certification Governance Committee. The following professionals served as members of the NLN's Certification Governance Committee:

Deborah Lindell, DNP, APRN, BC, CNE

Julia W. Aucoin, DNS, RN, BC, CNE

Carolyn E. Adams, EdD, RN, CNAA, BC

Maria A. Connolly, DNSc, APN/CNS, CNE, FCCM

Susan Devaney, EdD, APRN, BC

Annitta Love, MSN, RN

Nancy Sharts-Hopko, PhD, RN, FAAN

Mae E. Timmons, EdD, RN, CNE

Lin Zhan, PhD, RN, FAAN

Tracy A. Ortelli, MS, RN (NLN Manager, Academic Nurse Educator Certification Program)

The 2012 Revisions to this text were developed by the NLN CNE Task Group. The following professionals served as members of the 2012 Task Group:

Nancy Sharts-Hopko, PhD, RN, CNE, FAAN (CNE Commission Chair)

Marsha Adams, DSN, RN, CNE, ANEF

Pamela DiVito-Thomas, PhD, RN, CNE

Tara Hulsey, PhD, RN, CNE

Jan Nick, PhD, RN, CNE, ANEF

Judy K. Ogans, MS, RN, CNE

Linda S. Christensen, JD, MSN, RN (NLN Staff Liaison)

Ayana Nickerson (NLN Staff Liaison)

Larry E. Simmons, RN, PhD, CNE, NEA-BC (NLN Staff Liaison)

Final Thoughts

Nursing education is a dynamic field meeting the challenges of a nursing faculty shortage, increasingly sophisticated technologies, and the stimulation of a diverse student population. Clinical competence and educational expertise are required to continue the advancement of our specialty. The influence of evidence-based practice and new research in nursing education, the successful collaboration with other disciplines, and the mentorship of new faculty colleagues demand a dynamic and evolving scope of practice. The 2012 revision of *The Academic Scope of Practice for Academic Nurse Educators* reflects the dynamic evolution of the faculty role.

References

American Nurses Association. (2000). *Scope and standards of practice for nursing professional development.* Washington, DC: Author.

American Nurses Association. (2004). *Nursing: Scope and standards of practice.* Washington, DC: Author.

American Nurses Association. (2010). *Nursing's social policy statement: The essence of the profession.* Washington, DC: Author.

American Nurses Association. (2010). *Nursing: Scope and standards of practice, 2nd ed.* Washington, DC: Author.

Boyer, E. (1990). *Scholarship reconsidered: Priorities of the professoriate.* Princeton, NJ: The Carnegie Foundation for the Advancement of Teaching.

Caputi, L., & Engelmann, L. (2004). *Teaching nursing: The art and science.* Glen Ellyn, IL: College of DuPage Press.

Community Campus Partnerships for Health. (2004). Retrieved May 25, 2005 from http://depts.washington.edu/ccph/

Donahue, M.P. (1996). *Nursing, the finest art: An illustrated history* (2nd ed.). St. Louis: Mosby.

Fondiller, S. H. (1999). One hundred years ago: Nursing education at the dawn of the 20th century [From the archives]. *Nursing and Health Care Perspectives,* 20(6), 286-288.

Kalisch, P. & Kalisch, B. (1995). *The advance of American nursing* (3rd ed.). Philadelphia: J. B. Lippincott Co.

Kelly, L. Y., & Joel, L. A. (1996). *The nursing experience: Trends, challenges, and transitions* (3rd ed.). New York: McGraw-Hill.

Kirkpatrick, J., & Valley, J. (2004). Finding success in the faculty role. In L. Caputi, & L. Engelmann (Eds.), *Teaching nursing: The art and science.* Glen Ellyn, IL: College of DuPage Press, 972-989.

Knowles, M., Holton, E., & Swanson, R. (1998). *The adult learner: The definitive classic in adult education and human resource development* (5th ed.). Houston, TX: Gulf.

Kolb, D. A. (1984). *Experiential learning: Experience as a source of learning and development.* Englewood Cliffs, NJ: Prentice-Hall.

Krathwol, D. R., Bloom, B. S., & Masia, B. (1964). *Taxonomy of educational objectives, Handbook II.* New York: David McKay.

National League for Nursing (2002). Position Statement: The preparation of nurse educators. New York: National League for Nursing. Retrieved June 9, 2005 from www.nln.org/aboutnln/PositionStatements/prepofnursed02.htm

National League for Nursing (2004). *NLN Hallmarks of Excellence in Nursing Education.* New York: National League for Nursing. Retrieved July 19, 2012 from www.nln.org/excellence/hallmarks_indicators.htm

National League for Nursing. (2005a). *Core competencies of nurse educators.* New York: National League for Nursing. Retrieved June 9, 2005 from www.nln.org/profdev/corecompetencies.pdf.

National League for Nursing. (2005b). *Position statement: Transforming Nursing Education.* New York: National League for Nursing. Retrieved June 9, 2005 from www.nln.org/aboutnln/PositionStatements/transforming052005.pdf

National League for Nursing. (2005c). *The Scope of Practice for Academic Nurse Educators.* New York: National League for Nursing.

Tagliareni, M. E. & Marck, B. (1997). *Teaching in the community: Preparing nurses for the 21st century.* New York: National League for Nursing.